Lose 30 Pour
(Or Mc
Intermittei.. i ui.iii6 &
'Home' Coffee Enemas

CW00860211

Detoxify Your Body, Lose Weight, Get Healthy & Transform Your Life Volume 3

ROBERT DAVE JOHNSTON

Published by:

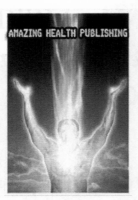

If you are interested in reading the next volume, follow Rob on Twitter @FitnessFasting

Copyright

Disclaimer & Legal Notices

The health-related information and suggestions contained in any of the books or written material mentioned above are based on the research, experience and opinions of the Author and other contributors. Nothing herein should be misinterpreted as actual medical advice, such as one would obtain from a Physician, or as advice for self-diagnosis or as any manner of prescription for self-treatment.

Neither is any information herein to be considered a particular or general cure for any ailment, disease or other health issue. The material contained within is offered strictly and solely for the purpose of providing Holistic health education to the general public. Persons with any health condition should consult a medical professional before entering this or any fasting, weight loss, detoxification or health related program.

Even if you suffer from no known illness, we recommend that you seek medical advice before starting any fasting, weight loss and/or detoxification program, and before choosing to follow any advice given this book. For any products or services mentioned or suggested in this book, you should read all packaging and instructions, as no substance, natural or drug, can be guaranteed to work in everyone. Information and statements regarding dietary supplements, products or services mentioned in this book many not have been evaluated by the Food and Drug Administration and are not intended to diagnose, treat, cure, or prevent any disease. Never disregard or delay in seeking professional medical advice because of something you have read in this book.

Nothing that you read in this book should be regarded as medical or health advice. If you do anything recommended in this book, without the supervision of a licensed medical doctor, you do so at your own risk. Not recommended for persons with any health related condition unless supervised by a qualified health practitioner.

Because there is always some risk involved in any health-related program, the Author, Publisher and contributors assume no responsibility for any adverse effects or consequences resulting from the use of any suggested preparations or procedures described in any of the books or other written materials associated with the website FitnessThroughFasting.com. The author reserves the right to alter and update his opinions based on new conditions at any time.

Dedication

This series of books are dedicated to my mother Sonia Noemi, without whom I would not even be alive today. I love you mom. Thank you for never losing faith in me and supporting me, even when everything seemed hopeless and everyone else had given up on me. I owe you everything. I could collect all of the precious stones on this earth and lay them on your lap, and even still, I would not even come close to giving back to you all that you have given me.

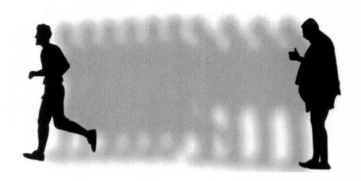

"From personal experience as well as that of others, you can expect to lose anywhere from 7-10 pounds weekly with this structure of intermittent fasting."

Chapter 1:
Rapid Weight Loss &
Detoxification

Without a doubt, the number one, most-asked question I receive about fasting is this – >

What is the Fastest Way to Lose Weight & Detoxify?

* If I had to narrow it down to two steps, these would be:

1) **Intermittent Fasting**

2) **Home "Coffee" Enemas**

I am assuming that you want to transform your life and health, not just put a little patch on the situation, right? • You want to: Lose weight & cleanse your body of harmful toxins that threaten your health and wellbeing. Gain knowledge that can **CONTINUALLY** help you maintain optimum weight and health. In think we can agree on those, right? So, let's talk about how to make it happen!

Intermittent Fasting

Intermittent fasting is practiced by many religions around the world. If you are a catholic, for example, you may be familiar with the way *"lent"* fasting is observed. To be sure, there are many different ways one can practice intermittent fasting.

But I don't want to bombard you with too much information. I want to draw a straight line from where you are now, to where you want to get. To simplify matters, we are going to refer to intermittent fasting as the practice of not eating from 10pm to 6pm each day, for 30 days.

20 Hours of Fasting Daily

This means that you will be fasting 20 hours daily, but will get to have dinner and a snack every night. You can do this for whatever period of time you wish.

However, for our purposes, we are sticking with the 30-day format for **maximum weight loss and detoxification**.

Water Fasting

During the day you will be water fasting. When I say water fasting, I mean that you will be drinking water only.

For 20 hours each day during the 30 days, you will eat no solid food, limiting yourself only to water

There is much wisdom and power to this practice. While with intermittent fasting the digestive system does not go into total hibernation as it happens during an extended water fast (*not eating for more than 72 hours*), the body still receives much-needed time to rest from the endless process of digestion.

This '*time off*' gives the digestive system the opportunity to focus on other important tasks such as detoxification, healing, tissue repair and, of course, rapid weight loss.

Lose Weight Fast

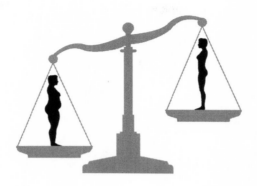

From personal experience as well as that of others, you can expect to lose anywhere from 7-10 pounds weekly from this type of intermittent fasting. I know of some people who have done this fast/detox program and lost in excess of 40, even 50 pounds.

I can't guarantee that you will lose that much weight. However, if you follow my instructions in detail, you will lose **A LOT** of weight for sure.

Alright – Let's Go!

Chapter 2:
Cut Out the Junk

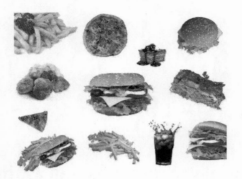

If you have been eating poorly and/or excessively, then I strongly advise you to go through a preparation phase of 7-10 days prior to starting. What do I mean by preparation?

Simply this: removing from your diet any and all junk, greasy and sugary foods that you are accustomed to eating.

The removal of these toxic foods will send your body into ultimate detoxification and fat-burning mode, so you will lose weight before you even begin fasting

Furthermore, a lot of the tougher toxins will be processed during those initial preparation days, meaning that the fasting detoxification symptoms will usually be less than if you didn't prepare at all. To keep matters simple, here is a list of the foods that you should avoid for 7-10 days before you start this program.

Banned Foods

*Salt - The foods we eat all have sodium. A healthy adult really has no need for 'salt' except to make the food taste better. When I stopped using salt, I immediately dropped 15 pounds. It was mostly water weight, but it showed me that I was retaining a **LOT** of liquids, and that was greatly due to my abuse of salt and seasonings.

Instead of salt, I have become accustomed to seasoning my food with garlic powder (*not garlic salt*), onion powder (*not onion salt*) and a few of the Ms. Dash no-salt seasonings. I don't even miss salt anymore. I can eat and enjoy food that, in the past, would have been totally bland. My taste buds have readjusted and I feel much better.

* **Sugar** - absolute trash, toxic to the body... good for nothing - stay away! I could write pages and pages about sugar. I am sure that you yourself can admit that this is one of our greatest (*if not our greatest*) enemy. I mean it. Enemy. Any prolonged return to sugar will, sooner or later, result in full-blown intoxication of the bloodstream and digestive system.

I don't kid myself by thinking that *"I'm cured."* I still am susceptible to sugar and binging. What keeps me free and clean is **NOT** to put sugar into my body... period.

I can't draw the same conclusion for you, but I am certain that you probably have your own stories to tell about sugar and how it has affected your weight, life and health.

* **Fried Foods** - Absolute filthy grease fest that leads to obesity and other diseases.

* **Cheese** - Cheese is delicious but is packed with fat. For the time being, steer clear. Later on, once you finish the fast and detox, you can decide what you wish to do.

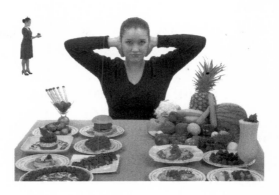

Don't let the mind start telling you that your *'life is over'* because you can't eat this or that. Just tell it to shut up. Keep moving forward.

* **Dairy Products** - dairy has a lot of fat, is high in sugar content and has been known to cause digestive system inflammation. But I'm not totally heartless. Stick to non-fat milk, how's that? Anything above non-fat is banned.

* **Red Meat** - I personally don't have anything against red meat. In fact, I have been known to eat a piece of meat on rare occasion. Right now, we are banning it because it has a lot of fat, and because I want your digestive system to be given easy food to digest.

15

Later on you can have a piece of meat here and there if you want. Right now... it's banned.

* **Alcohol** - Alcohol is packed with empty calories. Calories with **ZERO** nutritional value. And booze turns to sugar. Bad all over. If you drink frequently, cut it down to a minimum. You're doing this for your health and to reach a goal that is important to **YOU**.

If you have to go a few days without drinking, your arm is not going to fall off. You'll live. A cup of wine with dinner is fine, but nothing more than that at this juncture.

* **Butter or Margarine** - As they say in New York, "Forget about it!!!" Butter and margarine are pure fat and we don't want it.

* **Fruit Juices** - If you read the label of most orange juice brands, you will see that the sugar content is through the roof.

Yes, it is natural sugar, but sugar nonetheless. You can have one glass of juice in the morning, but you need to water it down 50/50.

Drinking straight juice at this phase is basically like injecting blubber directly into your belly. Stay away. **Drink veggie juice instead**...but make sure that it is the low sodium veggie juice.

***White Enriched Bread** - That stuff is like dropping a ball of cement into the stomach. White flour, doughy garbage really is terrible for human health. I was going to ban all breads, but I remembered that the Ezekiel brand (*green bag*) is actually very good. You can eat one slice here and there as partial replacement to your carbohydrate servings. We'll get into all of that in just a minute.

***Junk Food of <u>ANY</u> Kind** - I think that it definitely goes without saying that junk food is out. And not just out for a little while.

Hopefully, it is out of your life for good. That crap is like wearing a ball and chain. It enslaves us to cravings that are never satisfied and only get stronger and more violent.

Foods to Limit List:

*Fruits
(Stick To Strawberries or Cantaloupe)
* Tomatoes
* Peas or Corn
* Olive Oil

Starting immediately, eliminate **ALL** of these foods and beverages from your diet... period. This is the beginning of the process. For now, continue to eat whatever else you have been eating **EXCEPT** for the foods that are listed above. I want you to take a full step forward and discontinue eating any and all junk. That's the whole point of our work together, right? To help you achieve measurable improvements in your health. So cut it all out.

Do not eat even a little of them anymore. I mean Nothing, No More, Finito, Nada! You are taking the monumental step of removing **ALL** toxic foods from your diet. I use the word 'monumental' because, in truth, you are now in the minority. The majority of people live their whole lives and **NEVER** confront their eating behaviors as you are now doing. And since (*hopefully*) you won't be dumping more crap into your belly, the intermittent fasting and coffee enema cleanse will be able to go deep and discharge any hardened debris that hasn't come out via regular vowel movements.

You man now wonder: Ok, so what **CAN** I eat? To answer your question, let me show you my usual menu, which you can use as is, or arrange in similar fashion. The most important part of this preparation phase is that you steer clear of the 'banned foods' listed above. Do that and you will be on your way to amazing results with the actual fast and detox program.

Fail to do it, and you will bring upon yourself greater discomfort than you should, and – worse yet – the results will not be optimal.

So, please: Follow my instructions as closely as you possibly can. Trust me, **I have gone through this countless times and can tell you with certainty that preparation prior to fasting is absolutely indispensable.**

Chapter 3:
Sample Pre-Fasting Menu

As I said, you can use this menu exactly as written, or you can match it as close as possible. What matters most, once more, is that you observe the banned foods listed above. Follow this clean diet for at least 7 days before starting with intermittent fasting and coffee enemas. This is the path that will help you yield the best and most measurable results. The good news, however, is that the pre-fasting meal structure still allows you to eat generously; although – of course – there will be restrictions.

Sample Menu:

Breakfast 8:00 AM

1 Cup of Oatmeal with 1 Cup Skim Milk, a Handful of Raisins or Plums
Three Egg Whites mixed with, 3 OZ Ground Turkey
1 Cup of Green Tea with Stevia.

Mid-Morning Snack 10AM

1 Apple or Pear Mixed With One Cup of Nonfat Yogurt (*Plain*)
OR, ONE Apple, Pear, Banana or Other Fruit

Lunch - Noon

Big salad with lettuce, tomato and other veggies you may like. For dressing, use olive oil (no more than 1 teaspoon) and balsamic vinegar.1 Envelope of Low-Sodium Tuna
1 4OZ Baked Potato or Sweet Potato

Mid-Afternoon Snack 3PM

Same as before - I usually have a piece of fruit mixed with yogurt. At this time in the afternoon, I also drink another cup of green tea.

Green tea has energy-boosting and body-heating properties. It will help to give you a pep as well as calm hunger pangs. In addition to green tea, seltzer water (*sparkling water/club soda*) is great to navigate hunger.

Dinner - 6PM

Six-to-eight ounces of chicken, fish or ground turkey (*I like to make turkey patties*) Large salad as the one eaten for lunch. Steamed Broccoli, Cauliflower and Carrots (*most supermarkets have prepackaged vegetable combinations that are ready to steam and eat*).
4OZ Baked Potato or Sweet Potato **OR** 4OZ of Whole Wheat or Whole Grain Pasta **OR** 4 OZ of Brown Rice

Evening Snack - 8PM

Big salad with 3OZ Chicken, Fish or Ground Turkey - **No carbohydrates**. A piece of fruit with Non-fat Yogurt. Cup of Chamomile Tea - Chamomile tea is great to drink at night because it will help soothe hunger as well as calm you and get you ready for bed.

Note: You should not eat anything at least two hours prior to turning in, so time the final snack with your bedtime so that there the two-hour window is observed. I usually eat my last snack at around 10pm. Sometimes I also take one 500 mg tablet of Tryptophan at night to help me sleep.

Tryptophan is an awesome amino acid that helps to stabilize mood. At this point I'm done eating for the day and drink only water until 6PM the following evening.

Again ->

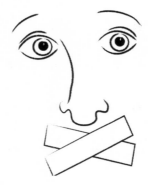

NEVER EAT FOR THE LAST TWO HOURS BEFORE YOU GO TO BED. TAPE YOUR MOUTH SHUT IF YOU HAVE TOO!

When the body is at rest, all of the metabolic processes slow down. You won't burn as many calories as you do during the day while you're moving around. When you eat large portions of food shortly before going to bed, many of those calories are directly stored as fat. In addition, rather than healing and restoring, the body spends the night digesting.

The end result, at least for me, is waking up feeling like a truck ran over me. Just slept eight hours, yet I feel tired, lethargic and irritable.

Bottom line:

Eating less than two hours before going to bed is a bad Idea. Tape your mouth shut if you have to. But eat no more!

Chapter 4:
Getting Started

Once you have completed the 7-10 days of preparation, you are ready to jump into the main part of this program. **<u>Do this</u>**:

• Pick the Day that you are going to start. Have your last regular meal the previous evening no later than 9 PM. Do not overeat thinking you are "*stuffing*" for the fast. That will only worsen the hunger pains and detox symptoms. In fact, that is precisely the reason why I asked you to do 7-10 days of preparation, so that your stomach will begin to shrink and start to require less foods to be satisfied.

• Start a **fasting journal** several days before you start. Include detailed writing on how much weight you want to lose and what your general goals are in this process. Write about your ideal body weight and the things you will do once you achieve it. A lot of people balk when I talk to them about starting a journal of any kind. I don't understand why.

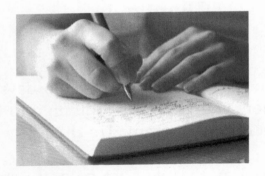

Keeping a journal of your goals, progress and challenges is one of the most powerful ways to ensure that you'll go the distance and achieve all of your objectives. There is nothing more powerful than reading your own reasons when you feel tired and wish to give up.

So, please – do it!

• Start your fast in the **AM** of the chosen day. Drink only water when the hunger pains hit you. Write on your journal if you start to feel angry, irritable or sad. These symptoms are normal and will pass as the days go by.

• If the hunger pains get really bad, try some seltzer/sparkling water with a small twist of lime. If this does not work, then drink more water and your stomach will be satisfied. Write on the fasting journal some more. Remind yourself why you are doing this and stick to your guns. And remind yourself that you will actually get to eat at the end of each day!

• Tell your belly to shut up. You are the boss of your body, not the other way around. Get angry with your stomach and *"literally"* tell it to be quiet and do as it is told. This sounds very silly but it has worked wonders for me. It has taught me that, in the end, I am the one who decides when and what to eat.

• At night, between 6 pm and 8 pm, eat a light meal made up mostly of poultry, fish, vegetables, brown rice and salad. Sugar and fried food of any type are strongly discouraged. Here's the meal that I usually have when I do this type of intermittent fast. It's the same one listed on the sample menu above. Make it as simple as possible so that, when nighttime comes, you don't find yourself wondering what you are going to eat. Plan ahead and make sure that you have everything that you will need to prepare the meals.

Dinner - 6PM

Six ounces of chicken, fish or ground turkey (*I like to make turkey patties*) Large salad and Steamed Broccoli, Cauliflower and Carrots (*most supermarkets have prepackaged vegetable combinations that are ready to steam and eat*). 4OZ Baked Potato or Sweet Potato OR 4OZ of Whole Wheat or Whole Grain Pasta OR 4 OZ of Brown Rice. For salad dressing, use a small dab of Olive Oil and a splash of Balsamic Vinegar.

Evening Snack - 8PM

Big salad with 3OZ Chicken, Fish or Ground Turkey - No carbohydrates. A piece of fruit with Non-fat Yogurt. Cup of Chamomile Tea.

As we discussed earlier, please do **NOT** eat anything else after your last snack.

The body needs those 12 hours of nightly fasting to process and expel all of the toxins that the coffee enemas will bring to the surface

• Keep a gallon of water next to your bed. If you wake up hungry in the middle of the night, take a large swig and go back to bed. If your bathroom happens to be next to the kitchen and you have to go, then go with blinders on –

DO_NOT_ by any means enter the kitchen for any reason whatsoever!

In The Morning

• Upon rising, have a large glass of water to stimulate the bowels. **Record on your journal how you are feeling physically and emotionally**. If you have any vivid or strange dreams, write about them. The release of large amounts of toxins into the bloodstream, as it occurs when fasting, can sometimes cause strange dreams. It is normal and will pass.

Fast the entire day following the steps described above.

• Carry out the coffee enema (*outlined below*) three times per week for the first two weeks, twice for the third week and once during the final week of the fast.

Monday, Wednesdays and Fridays are my personal choices.

• It is best to do the enema in the morning or, second best, at night **<u>BEFORE</u>** you break the fast with the evening meal.

• Make sure to read the instructions below several times so that you can learn to listen to your body and follow the protocol in a way that is best for your particular makeup and condition.

• On the last day of the fast, break it in the evening as usual.

Incorporate coffee enemas and 24-hour water fasting into your lifestyle at least <u>once per month</u>.

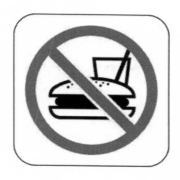

- **Most of all, do not return to consumption of damaging foods.** There's nothing worse than going through all of this work and sacrifice and then throwing a wrench in it by resuming a poor diet. It is my hope that, after this process, you will want to make permanent eating habit and lifestyle changes so that you can keep the benefits long term!

All told, you can lose from 30 to 50 pounds with this system, not to mention that you'll be ridding your body of disease-causing toxins & parasites.

Let's take a look at some of the detox symptoms that you may experience while fasting and cleansing.

Chapter 5:
Detox Symptoms

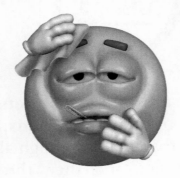

Headaches – This one is especially marked for coffee drinkers, but is also the case for persons who consume large amounts of sugar and alcohol. This symptom can really take a person out of commission.

A lot of my colleagues call me a heretic for saying this, but if you need to take a couple of ibuprofen tablets to ease the pain, then so be it. Usually two tablets will do the trick. But don't take more than four daily.

You may need to go through a little pain and discomfort. The good news is that headaches rarely last more than 72 hours, if that.

Dizziness – The body is not used to being deprived of eating whatever it wants and will go through dizzy spells, particularly during the first 11 days. The best solution for dizziness is to move slowly and get as much rest as your daily schedule allows.

Difficulty Performing Basic Tasks – Since you aren't consuming solid food, it will take some time for the body to adjust.

You will more than likely feel very weak and may have trouble getting around - particularly during the first 10-14 days. If you slow down and work on focusing on the individual tasks you are performing, this symptom can be overcome. It is important for you to realize that your body is going through a transition. You must move slowly and not try to push yourself too hard. You may not be able to function at the same capacity as you are accustomed. Fine. Slow down and give the body time to work on your behalf.

Weakness means that you need to be extra careful when walking around, and especially when getting up from a sitting position. Avoid harsh and/or abrupt movements.

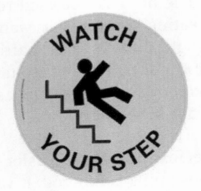

Move slowly, watch your step closely and always have something that you can hang on to if you suddenly feel like you are fainting. This is good advice.

One time I totally hit the deck because I got up to quickly from a chair. I missed the corner of the wall by centimeters, but still hit myself quite hard on the floor. This is about improving our health, not about getting hurt. Please be careful. I mean it. Be careful.

Pulsating Hunger Pains that disappear and then re-emerge throughout the day. For some persons, hunger is monstrous in the morning. But for the vast majority, the hunger troll shows up mostly at night.

In short, hunger will always be a part of our lives, and it is our task to master it rather than allow it to enslave us as it **CAN AND WILL** if we let it.

In my case, hunger was very strong in the first week to 10 days of intermittent fasting, and then I found myself getting used to always being 'a little' hungry.

After a while, I loved it because I began to feel more alert, more energetic, optimistic... I slept better. I actually **SLEPT THROUGH THE NIGHT** and woke up feeling terrific.

Before the fast, I constantly woke up at night to urinate, or like a raving lunatic wanting to raid the fridge. After a while, I would go to sleep at 11PM, close my eyes and, when I opened them, it was 6AM!

For me, this was nothing less than a total miracle. And I felt great... refreshed and ready to go! All of that just from getting used to eating less and being a little hungry.

Much better than getting stuffed like a boar as I used to.

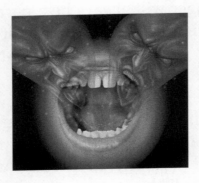

Bad Breath, Metallic Taste in Mouth, White Sticky Film on Tongue – These are all good indications that your body is eliminating toxicity.

Most of these symptoms pass after 14 days (*on average*). Bad Breath, I suggest that you get sugarless mints and keep them handy until the process ends.

Metallic Taste In the Mouth usually means that there are excessive (and toxic) heavy metals accumulated in your system.

I recall having this constant sulfur and 'steel' taste in my mouth for about a week.

White Sticky Film on the Tongue can be disgusting, but it's a sign that the body is cleansing.

For these symptoms, the best thing you can do is to keep drinking a lot of water. Make sure to brush your teeth regularly. Keep a travel toothbrush with you if you spend a lot of time out. Mouthwash is also helpful.

Diarrhea or Constipation – All of the fecal matter adhered to your colon will either start gushing out in diarrhea or incite short-term constipation. I know that this is disgusting, but it happens. If you have eaten poorly for a long time, or have simply abused sugar or fat, your body may respond to the water fast by starting to expel all of the toxic filth in this fashion.

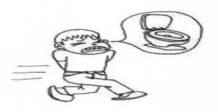

If **Diarrhea** Strikes, simply continue to follow the fast as outlined. Should it become severe, see your pharmacist and ask him or her for an over-the-counter recommendation.

Continue with the intermittent fast. **Fasting is a shock to the body, but it will finally get the message and react favorably to what you are doing.** If you have diarrhea, make sure to keep yourself hydrated.

Make it a point to drink at least <u>one gallon</u> of water daily. Stay close to a bathroom at all times. If you go out, make sure that you are always aware where the nearest restroom is. Seriously, you want to get to the toilet promptly anytime you need to.

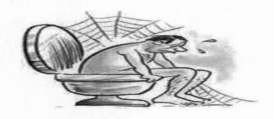

If **Constipation** is The Case, visit your local pharmacy and ask your pharmacist about a stool softener. I personally use a herbal laxative called <u>Herbs & Prunes</u>. It works like a charm every time and is not harsh on my stomach. Take one tablet to start. **Do not exceed four tablets in one day.** But do this only if you fail to eliminate anything for at least three days. Give your body enough time to do it on its own.

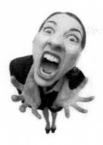

Irritability / Mood Swings – If you have ever seen The Flintstones, you may remember Fred walking around growling on the episode where he is placed on a diet.

Sooooo, be prepared to be a little *"short-fused"* during this time fasting and cleansing. Be aware that you will not be as patient as you normally would.

Tell your loved ones not to take it personally if - initially - you are less social that what they are accustomed. This is normal and will pass.

Facial Puffiness & Feeling Bloated – This symptom is much more marked for persons who consume large amounts of salt and/or sugar.

I was bloated to the max like the Stay Puft Marshmallow man (*pictured below*).

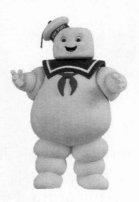

So being puffy was nothing new. I looked like somebody had stuck huge balloons on my cheeks. It was hideous. Fasting took care of that and my face today is that of a normal human being rather than a cartoon character.

That is a lot of symptoms, but rarely does **ONE** person experience them all. And remember, they will subside and mostly pass after approximately 14 days.

Continue to surrender to the process and stay put. Let the body do what it does best. Your body knows how to take care of you. Your body and digestive system thank you for this break.

Your body is loyal and noble ... it is unleashing amazing weight loss and healing power even as we speak. All you have to do is hang on and let the process run its course.

Chapter 6:
Coffee Enemas

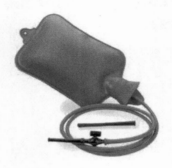

Yes, you heard right – I said Coffee enemas. This, without a doubt, is one of the most powerful detoxification tools I have discovered in my years as a fasting coach and practitioner. Caffeine incites stimulation of the digestive system which in turn induces what can often be dramatic elimination of toxic, hardened feces & parasites adhered to the walls of the colon.

If you look at the picture above, you can see the different conditions that can emerge when the colon is overloaded with toxins. And, trust me, you will be eliminating <u>a lot of gunk</u>. Even if you have eaten a clean diet, it is possible that you may still have substantial waste accumulated.

One man that I know eliminated pounds and pounds of undigested meat that was rotting in his colon!

Typically I am asked: *"Well, what is the difference between drinking coffee and a coffee enema?"*

Answer: "Drinking coffee often induces a bowel movement. This, effect, however is much deeper and thorough **when the coffee is injected directly into the colon rather than just as a beverage**. It is a very powerful colon detoxification technique."

Gross!

Now, when I start to talk about feces, parasites and enemas, many persons rapidly balk and become *"grossed out,"* indicating that they are not interested in anything that has to do with "rectal insertion."

They are, in essence, horrified by the prospect. You would think one is asking them to sever a limb or something.

My response is always the same:

"Well, would you rather be a little grossed out and rid your body of these derelict parasites and toxins <u>NOW</u>, or would you prefer to deal with them <u>LATER</u> in a hospital bed or – god forbid – with a life-threatening illness?"

If you are one of these persons, I hope this response helps to put things in perspective.

Believe me, whatever feeling of *"grossness"* you feel is small in comparison to the huge health benefits this practice can offer. Ok, so how is this done?

<u>Do this</u>: Go to your local pharmacy and/or health store and purchase a <u>One Gallon Enema Kit</u> at the very minimum.

In addition, purchase a bag of surgical gloves, as well as some Vaseline or other lubricant **AND** rubbing alcohol.

One you have the enema kit, gloves, alcohol and lubricant on hand, it's time to prepare the coffee solution and get started.

Preparing the Coffee Solution

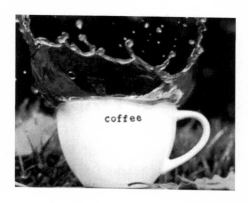

In terms of which type of coffee to use, the truth is that it doesn't really matter so long as it is caffeinated, of course. I use either **Maxwell House or Café Bustelo**. They both do the job quite well.

But you can safely use whatever coffee you are used to drinking. What we're after is the caffeine in the liquid. I have not found any particular brand to work better than another.

Follow this step-by-step-approach:

• The night before, brew at least 2 full pots of coffee – equivalent to 12 cups in most coffee makers. Use 10 table spoons of coffee for each brewing.

• Place each yield of coffee in a large soup pan for cooling. If you don't have a large pan, you may need to use several smaller ones. The point is that you pour the coffee into a separate recipient for cooling.

• Take at least 3 empty water gallons and fill each *"halfway"* with filtered or purified water. I strongly discourage the use of tap water.

Fill the rest of the gallon with the cooled coffee. Continue this process until you have filled at least <u>three</u> gallons of the coffee/water mixture. This should last you one week.

Getting It Done

• When you are ready, go to your bathroom and place various towels on the floor next to the door, as well as two pillows. I also bring in a <u>portable radio and put on soothing music for relaxation</u>.

• Assemble the enema bag with the enclosed hook for the top, the hose and *"inserter"* at the bottom. Make sure the enema "lock" is closed.

Pour some water on the enema bag and make sure that it is not leaking and that the lock is properly in place.

• Many enema hoses have various "lock" positions that go from zero, to small, to large releases of liquid.

Get acquainted with the one you have and learn how to go from little to more water with each different lock position. Learn exactly where the "total lock" position is.

• Play with the hose for a few minutes until you feel comfortable with it and understand how to regulate the levels of liquid that it releases. If the one you have only goes from lock to release, observe the amount of liquid that comes out when it is open.

The point is, see what you are working with **NOW**. Once you are on the floor and using it, you do not want any surprises.

• When all looks good, dump the "test" water and fill the enema bag with the coffee/water mixture. Carry the enema bag to the bathroom through the plastic hook at the top (*enclosed with the enema*).

• Hang the enema bag in the bathroom door knob. I use the door knob because it grants enough slack between the hose and body.

Experiment in your bathroom and find the most comfortable location for the bag. Make sure the enema bag is steady and that it will not fall wherever you decide to place it.

• Next, wash your hands thoroughly with hot water. Use germ-killing bar or liquid soap. Scrub all the way up your forearms like a surgeon before surgery.

• Turn off all telephones and, if you live with others, make sure that you inform them not to disturb you.

• Next, put on the sterilized plastic gloves. Get the Vaseline and lubricate the "inserter" tip of the enema.

• Lay down sideways on the floor, your head on one of the pillows and your back facing the enema bag. Depending on which side you lay, grab the inserter with your free hand. It is now time to do the deed.

• Slowly spread some lubricant around your rectum. Little by little, insert the tip of the enema inside of you. Take your time. Do not force it in. If it feels dry and painful, take it out and put more lubricant. Repeat this process until you are able to insert it without undue pain.

• Once in, reach to the enema bag lock. Take a deep breath and release the lock so that it starts to let out the smallest amount of the coffee/water mixture. You will feel the cool liquid start to enter your belly.

• Let the liquid continue to enter your colon for at least ten seconds. Lock the hose and make sure the surge of liquid has stopped.

• Begin to massage your stomach from different angles. At this point you may or may not get the urge to eliminate. If you do, try to hold it - if you can. If not, then go ahead and eliminate.

• If you **CAN** hold it, then "open" the lock again for another ten seconds, this time so that it releases a larger amount of the coffee/water mixture.

• Once you feel your colon is pretty full of the mixture, remove the inserter from your rectum, wrap it in toilet paper and set it aside.

•Lay face up with one pillow under your head and another one under your lower back.

Massaging the Belly

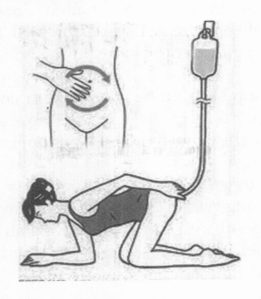

It is now that the real work begins. Spend as much time as possible massaging your stomach with both hands –> covering the left, right, bottom and upper parts of your abdomen. Pay close attention to your liver.

Let the music sink in and visualize toxins, parasites and hardened feces being expelled from your body. Take as much time as needed in this process. Really, really work it!

For some persons with large levels of toxicity, the evacuation process can be dramatic and almost immediate. If that is the case for you, go ahead and eliminate. You may feel cramps in your stomach and some abdomen pain. This is fairly normal for most people. Make sure to look at the discharge once you are done. What color is it? Is it really dark or even black? If so, then it is likely that you are making good progress.

If at any time you see blood in the stool, stop the enema immediately and go see your doctor at once! Repeat this method until the mixture in the enema bag is consumed.

If the evacuation does not instantly come, persist with the massage. If there is still no discharge, go ahead and eliminate and repeat the process. You may have very hardened or stubborn buildup in your bowels.

Chapter 7:
Take Your Time

For me, the process was very slow. I actually would fill my colon with the mixture, get up and go about other business around the house, keeping the liquid inside of me for several hours at a time. It may take time for the dregs of fecal matter to soften and be expelled. Don't give up! So, if you are the type who is slow to discharge, get up and do something else. But please, stay close to a bathroom at all times! Let's avoid embarrassing accidents!

Adjusting the Coffee Mix

Use up the entire contents of the enema bag during the day. I recommend you do the whole bag in one session. But, if you are pressed for time, **it is okay to do part in the morning and the rest at night – so long as you do not use the same mixture**! Dump any unused mixture at once; do not store it for later use, please. If you find that the current mixture is not working, prepare another one with more coffee.

Go from, say, 10 tablespoons of coffee per pot to 15.

Keep trying until you find your magic number. For some people who are obese and highly toxic, as many as 20 tablespoons of coffee per pot (*or more*) may be required. Take it slow and continue the process until you find the right formula for you. But do not overdo it with the coffee! It is best to start low and go up gradually. If you add too much coffee, you may get very painful and uncomfortable cramps. Don't make it any harder than it has to be, please!

When you are done, make sure to wash the inserter with hot water and soap, **<u>AND</u>** dip it into a small cup filled with rubbing alcohol. Do this with the gloves still on. Wash the enema bag in warm water with the hose "open" so that it cleanses the inside of it as well. Hang it to dry. I hang mine in the shower curtain bar.

Be very thorough with the inserter and make sure it is painstakingly clean and sterilized. Once done, wrap it again in toilet paper and put it away with the enema bag as described below.

Make sure you store the enema kit where others will **NOT** have access to it.

NEVER share the inserter with anybody else no matter how clean it is. In fact, don't share the enema bag at all.

Let each family member interested in fasting and cleansing purchase one of their own. Pick up the towels from the floor and put them in the washer, along with the pillow cases from the pillows you used during the process.

Once the enema bag is dry, I recommend you store it in a "zip-lock" bag along with the inserter. That way your kit will not be exposed to dust, germs or any type of dirt. If you need to mop the bathroom because some liquid spilled, do so **BUT** keep the gloves on.

Bleach the bathroom floor as well as the toilet. When you are done, THEN remove the gloves and throw them out. Go through the initial hand-washing process again and finalize by sprinkling them with rubbing alcohol. Allow hands to air dry.

If you have children, **DO NOT** dispose the gloves by simply throwing them on top of the garbage pail. One of the little-ones may reach in and retrieve them! On the next session, wash each part of the kit thoroughly and again sterilize the inserter with rubbing alcohol.

The bottom line is this: with intermittent fasting combined with coffee enemas, you will experience very rapid weight loss as well as the deep cleansing of your bowels.

This combination is extremely powerful. If you take the time to really get good at it, you will truly revolutionize your health. It may take some time to see the huge results that you seek, but if you are persistent, I can assure you that they will come.

Be patient and kind to your body, and it will pay you back in spades – guaranteed. In addition to discharging a lot of toxic muck from your bowels, you will start to feel lighter, more energetic, with greater mental energy and clarity. I know of people who found relief from chronic depression and other mental illnesses via coffee enemas and intermittent fasting.

If you stick to the plan for the 30 days, tremendous things will come to pass in your life and health. To finalize, here's a motivational message that I want you to keep in mind as you move forward.

Chapter 8:
The Challenge of
Detoxification

If you stumbled and were not able to complete the entire fast/cleansing, please don't worry. Yes, I know – it is a tough call. But it is not impossible. If you carried out the diet menu as outlined (*I strongly encourage you to do so*), then you now have a very good idea of the symptoms to expect when you try again.

So... just because you fell short of the goal and were unable to complete the fast/cleanse in one or multiple attempts, that does not mean that you failed. Such distinction is crucial because it is at this point that many give up.

They feel that going the distance is too hard and not feasible. Nothing is further from the truth. It may take a few attempts, but if you continue and not give up, you will make amazing progress. I was a complete disaster; obese, a food addict, depressed and suicidal... yet after some tries I **DID** complete the 30-day fast/cleanse. I would dare to say that I owe my life to it. So there is no way that you can fail.

You are continuing to learn and position yourself for breakthrough. This process is challenging but highly rewarding. So do not be discouraged. Progress, not perfection – is the key!

Keep the Journal Alive

Write, write and write as much as you can! Keep putting your thoughts and feelings on paper. Read this book several times until you feel that you have fully internalized the material.

If you truly are committed to change and find yourself struggling, then **it is fine to move at your own pace**. Stick to the program and keep working.

Try, try again. Take notes and learn from your mistakes. Your desire / willingness to change **WILL** help you to produce the breakthrough you want **IF** you stick to it. You can do it!

When tempted to stray, always remember:
Nothing Tastes as Good as Thin Feels!

God bless and Godspeed,

ROBERT DAVE JOHNSTON

Grab The Entire Collection:

Volume 1: The 'Permanent Weight Loss' Diet

Volume 2: The Intermittent Fasting Weight Loss Formula

Volume 3: How to Lose 30 Pounds (Or More) In 30 Days with Juice Fasting

Volume 4:_Lose The Belly Fat Fast, And For Good!

Volume 5: Lose the Emotional Baggage: Transform Your Mind & Spirit with Fasting

Volume 6: How to Break a Fast (or Diet) and Keep the Weight Off

Volume 7: Compilation Volumes 1-6 -> Get All 5 For The Price Of 3!

Also by Robert Dave Johnston:

How to Lose Weight & Keep it Off by Transforming the Mind & Behaviors

Volume 1: How to Build a Rock-Solid Foundation That Supports Long-Term Weight Loss

Volume 2: How to Lose Weight & Keep it Off By Reprogramming the Subconscious Mind

Volume 3: How to Beat Diet Hunger and Junk Food Cravings

Volume 4: How to Escape the Diet "Time Trap" and Succeed in Weight Loss

Volume 5: How to Cheat on Your Diet (And Get Away With It)

Volume 6, Compilation: All 5 for the Price Of 3

Also By Robert Dave Johnston:

Detoxify Your Body, Lose Weight, Get Healthy & Transform Your Life

Volume 1- The 10-Day 'At Home' Colon Cleansing Formula

Volume 2- The 30-Day Kidney, Parasite & Liver Detox Weight Loss Method

Volume 3- Lose Weight Fast & Detoxify With Intermittent Fasting & At-Home Coffee Enemas

Volume 4 - Compilation: Get All 3 For The Price Of 2! Detoxify Your Body, Lose Weight, Get Healthy & Transform Your Life - Volumes 1-3

Don't forget to check the articles and growing health community at: FitnessThroughFasting.com

Printed in Great Britain
by Amazon.co.uk, Ltd.,
Marston Gate.